UNDERSTANDING PROGERIA

A Comprehensive Guide to Understanding, Navigating, and Thriving with Progeria

Rachel J. Oles

<u>Table of Contents</u>

Chapter 1

<u>OVERVIEW OF PROGERIA SYNDROME</u>

Progeria (pro-JEER-e-uh), usually known as Hutchinson-Gilford progeria syndrome, is an extraordinarily rare, progressive hereditary condition. It causes youngsters to mature swiftly, starting in their first two years of life.

Children with progeria often appear healthy at birth. During the first year, indications such as slowed growth, loss of fat tissue, and hair loss begin to appear.

There are several forms of progeria, but the fundamental variety is known as Hutchinson-Gilford progeria syndrome (HGPS).

Children with this condition live on average for 14 years, because of the likelihood of developing atherosclerosis.

Around the world, 134 youngsters are thought to have progeria in 46 countries. It is projected to afflict 1 in every 4 million trustworthy Source infants of both sexes and all ethnicities.

Thirty years ago, little was understood about the cause of progeria. In 2003, a progeria gene was discovered. This has brought optimism that a solution might one day be found.

It is sometimes termed "Benjamin Button disease," after Scott Fitzgerald's fictional figure. However, in the story, "The Curious Case of Benjamin Button," Fitzgerald's character ages backward. People with progeria age ahead yet fast.

<u>SYMPTOMS OF PROGERIA</u>

1. <u>Growth Failure:</u> One of the early symptoms of progeria is a failure to thrive in infancy. Babies with progeria may have inadequate weight gain and growth, resulting in lower stature relative to their contemporaries.

2. <u>Premature Ageing:</u> Progeria causes the affected child's body to age fast, resulting in the appearance of features normally associated with old age. This premature ageing includes:
- Wrinkled and aged-looking skin.
- Prominent veins and visible blood vessels.
- Loss of subcutaneous fat, creating a thin and haggard appearance.

3. <u>Alopecia (Hair Loss):</u> Individuals with progeria often experience severe hair loss, which can occur on the scalp, eyebrows, and eyelashes.

4. <u>Aged Appearance of the Face:</u> The face may show a characteristic appearance, including:
- A tiny and pinched nose.
- A retreating chin.
- A narrow upper lip.
- Protruding ears.

5. <u>Joint Stiffness and Limited Range of Motion:</u> Progeria can lead to joint stiffness and contractures, decreasing the affected person's mobility and range of motion.

6. <u>Cardiovascular Abnormalities:</u> The most serious and life-threatening symptom of progeria is cardiovascular issues. Affected persons have an increased likelihood of getting heart disease and may experience symptoms such as:
- High blood pressure (hypertension).
- Narrowing of blood vessels (atherosclerosis).
- Hardening of the arteries (arteriosclerosis).

- Heart murmurs.
- Heart failure.

7. <u>Delayed and Poor Dentition:</u> Children with progeria may have delayed tooth eruption and dental difficulties, including crowding of teeth and thin tooth enamel.

8. <u>Fragile Bones:</u> Progeria can lead to weakened bones, making affected individuals more susceptible to fractures.

9. <u>Weariness and Muscle Weakness:</u> Individuals with progeria may develop muscle weakness, which can contribute to weariness and poorer physical endurance.

CAUSES AND GENETICS OF PROGERIA

Progeria, specifically Hutchinson-Gilford Progeria Syndrome (HGPS), is an unusual genetic disorder caused by a spontaneous mutation in the LMNA gene.

The LMNA gene encodes the lamin A protein, which plays a key function in preserving the structural integrity of the cell nucleus. Progeria is defined by the manufacture of an abnormal protein named progerin, which derives from a point mutation in the LMNA gene.

1. <u>Genetic Mutation:</u> The Mutation Responsible for Progeria. Progeria is primarily caused by a point mutation in the LMNA gene. This mutation comprises a single nucleotide modification in the DNA sequence, leading to the erroneous splicing of the pre-mRNA transcript. As a consequence, an aberrant and shorter variant of lamin A, known as progerin, is generated.

2. <u>Spontaneous Mutation:</u> De Novo Mutation. The vast majority of cases of progeria are the consequence of de novo mutations, meaning they emerge

spontaneously during the development of egg or sperm cells. These mutations are not inherited from the parents but develop through chance. Progeria is not related to any specific ethnic group or geographic region, and it occurs at a similar frequency in various people globally.

3. <u>Autosomal Dominant Inheritance:</u> While most occurrences of progeria come from de novo mutations, in rare occasions, the mutation could be inherited from one of the parents. Progeria follows an autosomal dominant inheritance pattern, which suggests that only one copy of the mutant gene (LMNA) is essential to produce the disorder. In such instances, affected individuals have a parent with the same genetic mutation.

4. <u>The Role of Progerin in Cellular Dysfunction:</u> Progerin impairs the regular operation of the cell nucleus and has severe repercussions on several cellular processes.

It leads to structural irregularities inside the nucleus, causing the nucleus to become deformed and unstable. This instability contributes to the accelerated ageing of affected cells and tissues.

5. <u>Cellular Ageing and Progeria:</u> Progeria is usually referred to as a segmental progeroid disorder, as it resembles some aspects of the normal ageing process. However, it is crucial to underline that progeria and normal ageing are distinct phenomena, with different underlying causes. The accelerated ageing seen in progeria is a result of the specific genetic mutation and the creation of progerin.

6. <u>Role of Lamin A Protein in Healthy Cells:</u> In healthy cells, lamin A performs a critical job in preserving nuclear integrity, controlling gene expression, and sustaining the overall structure of the cell nucleus. It forms part of the nuclear lamina, a protein

network that lines the inner surface of the nuclear envelope.

7. <u>Additional Progeroid Syndromes:</u> Apart from HGPS, there are additional progeroid syndromes caused by mutations in other genes. These syndromes may have some clinical signs with progeria but are independent disorders with different genetic causes. Some examples of other progeroid syndromes include Werner syndrome and Restrictive Dermopathy.

8. <u>Advances in Research:</u> Over the years, extensive work into the genetics of progeria has led to a clearer awareness of the disorder. Scientists continue to research the underlying mechanisms of progeria, searching for novel therapeutic targets and treatments. Recent developments in gene editing and targeted treatments give promise for potential future solutions.

How long do progeria patients live?
Progeria causes early death. People with the condition usually only live to their teenage years (average lifetime of 14 years). However, some can live into their early 20s. The cause of death is very often related to the heart or a stroke.

What kills people with progeria?
Hutchinson-Gilford progeria syndrome (HGPS) is an extraordinarily rare disease distinguished by the rapid appearance of ageing beginning in youth. Serious cardiovascular disorders can be life-threatening events for affected persons and cause early death.

Who is most prone to have progeria?
The disease affects folks of all sexes and races equally. About 1 in every 4 million newborns are born with it worldwide.

Is progeria more common in males than females?

Progeria is an extremely rare condition with typical clinical signs of early and accelerated ageing. Its incidence was anticipated to be one per eight million live births in the United States. Male to female ratio is around 1.5 -- 1.

Hutchinson-Gilford Progeria Syndrome is an extremely rare and dangerous hereditary disorder distinguished by accelerated ageing and concomitant health concerns. Its unusual features have motivated extensive research efforts, resulting in a deeper grasp of the genetic roots and molecular mechanisms involved in this condition.

While there is yet no cure for HGPS, the development of novel therapeutic procedures shows promise for improving the lives of affected persons and their families.

Chapter 2

<u>HISTORY AND TYPES OF PROGERIA</u>

Hutchinson-Gilford Progeria Syndrome (HGPS), generally known as progeria, is an extraordinarily rare and fatal hereditary disorder distinguished by rapid and premature ageing of affected individuals.

The condition was first described by Dr. Jonathan Hutchinson in 1886 and later by Dr. Hastings Gilford in 1904. HGPS is one of the most well-known and studied progeroid syndromes, generating great interest from the medical profession and the public due to its unusual and devastating features.

1. Clinical Features of HGPS:
HGPS presents with a distinct set of clinical symptoms, which become visible in the first

year of birth but are usually most noticeable throughout early childhood. The most characteristic indicators of HGPS include:

- <u>Growth Failure:</u> Affected individuals endure a failure to flourish, resulting in a substantially decreased height and weight relative to their contemporaries.

- <u>Premature Ageing of the Skin:</u> The skin of people with HGPS becomes thin, wrinkled, and aged in appearance. It may also show indications of pigmentation abnormalities.

- <u>Alopecia:</u> Progressive hair loss, especially on the scalp, eyebrows, and eyelashes, is a typical symptom of HGPS.

- <u>Facial Characteristics:</u> Affected individuals have a peculiar facial look, including a small and pinched nose, a receding chin, narrow lips, and projecting ears.

- <u>Cardiovascular Complications:</u> HGPS is related to a high risk of cardiovascular problems, such as atherosclerosis, which can lead to heart attacks and strokes at an early age.

- <u>Skeletal Abnormalities:</u> Children with HGPS may have skeletal abnormalities, including joint stiffness, limited range of motion, and hip dislocation.

2. Genetic Basis of HGPS:

The primary aetiology of HGPS depends on a unique spontaneous mutation in the LMNA gene, which encodes the lamin A protein. This mutation involves a single nucleotide change in the gene's DNA sequence, resulting in the synthesis of an abnormal protein named progerin.

Progerin impairs the proper activity of the cell nucleus and generates structural abnormalities, contributing to the accelerated ageing of damaged cells and tissues.

3. Impact on Cellular Function:

Progerin disrupts the architecture of the cell nucleus, leading to cellular dysfunctions that impede various key activities. Cells in patients with HGPS display greater genomic instability and senescence, contributing to the ageing process.

The presence of progerin affects the structural integrity of the nuclear envelope, leading to nuclear blebbing and deformed nuclei.

4. Cardiovascular Complications:

The most significant characteristic of HGPS is its link with cardiovascular issues. Atherosclerosis, characterised by the formation of fatty deposits in the arteries, is a key hallmark of HGPS.

The vascular system's premature ageing elevates the risk of heart attacks and strokes in affected individuals, primarily during their adolescent years.

5. Cognitive and Intellectual Development:

It's crucial to stress that HGPS does not affect cognitive or intellectual development. Individuals with HGPS typically have normal intelligence and cognitive abilities, however, they may meet hurdles pertaining to physical limits and health concerns.

6. Impact on Families and Research:

The diagnosis of HGPS has considerable emotional and practical repercussions for afflicted families. It often leads to a search for answers, support, and engagement in research efforts aimed at understanding and potentially treating progeria.

The Progeria Research Foundation (PRF) has been at the forefront of advancing research and promoting awareness of HGPS worldwide.

TYPES

Atypical Progeria Syndromes, sometimes known as progeroid syndromes, is a collection of rare genetic conditions that share certain similarities with Hutchinson-Gilford Progeria Syndrome (HGPS), but have unique genetic causes and clinical manifestations.

These disorders are characterised by signs of accelerated ageing and may emerge with diverse health concerns. Although they are separate illnesses from HGPS, they belong within the broader group of progeroid disorders due to their overlapping clinical features. Here are some instances of atypical progeria syndromes:

<u>Werner Syndrome (WS)</u>

Werner syndrome, generally known as adult progeria, is an autosomal recessive condition caused by mutations in the WRN gene, discovered on chromosome 8.

This gene encodes a helicase protein involved in DNA repair and maintenance. Individuals with Werner syndrome frequently appear healthy at birth but start showing symptoms of fast ageing in late adolescence or early adulthood. Some prominent elements of Werner syndrome include:

- Premature greying and loss of hair.
- Thinning and stiffened skin contribute to a characteristic "bird-like" aspect.
- Cataracts and eyesight difficulties.
- An increased risk of age-related illnesses, such as diabetes, atherosclerosis, and some cancers.
- Short stature and osteoporosis.

- Joint stiffness and limited mobility.

Restrictive Dermopathy (RD)

Restrictive dermopathy is an exceptionally rare and severe progeroid disorder caused by mutations in the ZMPSTE24 gene. This gene encodes a protein involved in the conversion of prelamin A to lamin A.

Defective processing of prelamin A resulted in the development of farnesyl-prelamin A, leading to nuclear abnormalities. Affected individuals usually do not live past the neonatal stage and may have the following features:

- Tight, tight, and thin skin with a shiny sheen.
- Joint contractures and reduced motion.
- Respiratory and nutrition difficulties.
- Failure to blossom and development retardation.
- Cardiovascular abnormalities.

<u>Nestor-Guillermo Progeria Syndrome (NGPS)</u>

Nestor-Guillermo Progeria Syndrome is another rare form of progeria caused by mutations in the BANF1 gene. Individuals with NGPS may have certain qualities with HGPS, including accelerated ageing and cardiovascular problems, but may have unique clinical presentations. Research into NGPS is ongoing, and its specific features and natural history are currently being researched.

It is crucial to emphasise that each atypical progeria syndrome is a separate genetic disorder, and the underlying mutations influence various genes and cellular processes.

As with HGPS, atypical progeria syndromes have no cure, and treatment mainly focuses on treating symptoms and promoting quality of life. Early diagnosis and thorough medical therapy, frequently involving numerous medical specialists, can help address specific health concerns and provide support to afflicted individuals and their families.

Furthermore, studying the genetics and biology of atypical progeria syndromes contributes to a greater understanding of ageing-related processes and may offer insights into possible therapy techniques for progeroid disorders. Research in this field continues to develop, presenting hope for enhanced care and perhaps personalised therapies in the future.

Chapter 3

CHALLENGES OF LIVING WITH PROGERIA

Living with progeria, specifically Hutchinson-Gilford Progeria Syndrome (HGPS), poses enormous hurdles for affected individuals and their families.

Progeria is an exceptionally rare and progressive hereditary disorder defined by early ageing, and the issues it provides are distinct and wide-ranging. Here are some of the primary concerns experienced by persons living with progeria:

1. Physical restrictions: Progeria generates severe physical limits due to the rapid ageing of tissues and organs. Affected patients typically feel joint stiffness, limited mobility, and skeletal abnormalities, which

can make daily tasks, such as walking, dressing, and eating, harder.

2. <u>Cardiovascular difficulties:</u> The most life-threatening component of progeria is its association with cardiovascular issues. Atherosclerosis, the formation of fatty deposits in the arteries, can lead to heart attacks and strokes at an early age. Managing cardiovascular health and monitoring heart function are crucial but demanding components of living with progeria.

3. <u>Growth Failure and Developmental Delays:</u> Children with progeria may experience growth failure, resulting in reduced stature and delayed physical development. Developmental deficits, including delayed tooth eruption and speech difficulties, may also be present.

4. <u>Nutritional and Dietary Challenges:</u> Maintaining a nutritious and balanced diet

might be an issue for persons with progeria. They may require unique dietary strategies to meet their nutritional needs and address growth and weight concerns.

5. <u>Increased Susceptibility to Infections:</u> Progeria affects the immune system, making affected patients more prone to infections. Simple infections might grow severe and require immediate medical intervention.

6. <u>Emotional and Psychological Struggles:</u> Coping with a rare and life-limiting condition like progeria can take an emotional toll on afflicted individuals and their families. The problems of living with a developing and visibly recognizable disease may add to feelings of isolation and low self-esteem.

7. <u>Social and Peer connections:</u> Children with progeria may have trouble in social connections because of their distinctive features and physical limitations. Educating

peers, teachers, and the community about progeria can help create a more inclusive and supportive environment.

8. <u>Financial and Accessible Healthcare Concerns:</u> The expert medical care required for controlling progeria can be costly and tricky to access, especially for families without enough financial resources or living in places with limited healthcare facilities.

9. <u>End-of-Life Planning:</u> Due to the progressive nature of progeria, affected patients and their families may need to address end-of-life planning and palliative care alternatives, which can be exceedingly distressing for all concerned.

10. <u>Coping with Loss:</u> Progeria has a considerable impact on life expectancy, with most individuals not enduring past their teenage years. Coping with the loss of a loved one due to progeria is a horrible reality experienced by families.

11. <u>Educational and Academic hurdles:</u> Children with progeria may have specific educational hurdles due to physical limits, developmental delays, and potential absences from school for medical treatments. Adapting the learning environment to match their requirements and giving additional educational support may be necessary to ensure academic progress.

12. <u>Health Monitoring and Medication Management:</u> Living with progeria involves regular medical check-ups and vigilant monitoring of several health markers. Managing medications, therapies, and therapeutic interventions can be tough for both individuals with progeria and their caretakers.

13. <u>Alter Family ties:</u> Progeria can radically alter the relationships inside a family. Caregivers may confront increased responsibility in delivering physical and

emotional aid, while siblings may experience a combination of emotions, including concern for their affected brother or sister, and feelings of being forgotten or abandoned.

14. <u>Accessibility and Inclusivity:</u> Public locations, transportation, and buildings may not always be entirely accessible to persons with physical restrictions, especially those with progeria. Ensuring inclusion and accessibility in many settings can enhance the quality of life and social participation for persons with progeria.

15. <u>Advocacy and Awareness:</u> Families of individuals with progeria often become advocates for their loved ones and promote awareness about the condition to increase understanding and support within their communities. Advocacy initiatives serve a key role in furthering research, giving access to services, and establishing a feeling of community among affected families.

16. <u>Emotional Support and Mental Health:</u> Living with progeria can provoke a range of feelings, including tension, anxiety, and grief. Access to mental health treatment and counselling is vital for individuals with progeria and their families to manage the emotional issues that accompany the condition.

17. <u>Limited Treatment Options:</u> As of today, there is no cure for progeria. The rarity of the illness and the intricacy of its underlying genetic pathways provide problems in designing targeted treatments. Continued research efforts and clinical trials are required to examine potential therapy options.

Living with progeria poses a complex set of issues for affected persons and their families. However, with a mix of medical care, emotional support, advocacy efforts, and a sense of community, persons with progeria can find resilience and strength.

Research and improvements in healthcare continue to bring promise for improved management and future treatments, ultimately boosting the quality of life for persons living with progeria and their families.

Chapter 4

<u>PROGERIA AND SCHOOL</u>

Navigating school and education when you have progeria can offer unique issues related to physical limits, significant developmental delays, and the need for specialised care.

However, with careful planning, collaboration between parents, educators, and medical professionals, and a supportive school environment, persons with progeria can have a happy and meaningful educational experience. Here are some essential concerns for addressing school and education when living with progeria:

1. Individualised Education Plan (IEP):

Developing an Individualised Education Plan (IEP) is crucial for students with progeria. An IEP outlines specialised goals, adjustments, and support services to suit the individual requirements of the student. This plan may include changes to the curriculum, assistive technology, prolonged breaks, or flexible scheduling to accommodate medical visits.

2. Early Communication with School Staff:

It is vital to communicate early with the school administration, instructors, and support professionals about the student's condition and particular requirements. Educating school staff about progeria helps foster a clearer understanding of the challenges the student confronts and ensures that suitable adjustments are in place.

3. Physical Accessibility:

Ensuring physical accessibility within the school premises is critical for students with progeria. This involves installing ramps, elevators, accessible amenities, and classrooms located on the ground floor to accommodate mobility concerns.

4. Medical Care and Emergency Preparedness:

Schools should have a complete awareness of the student's medical needs and a plan for managing any crises that may develop. Training school personnel in basic medical procedures, such as CPR, and giving them information about the student's medical condition can be important in emergency situations.

5. Flexible Learning Environments:

Offering a flexible learning environment can allow individuals with progeria to thrive academically. This may include flexible seating, access to technology, and the ability for remote study during times when the student's health requires it.

6. Emotional and Social Support:

Students with progeria may face emotional and social challenges due to their physical appearance and limitations. Providing a supportive and inclusive school climate that emphasises empathy, kindness, and awareness can assist adolescents with progeria to feel welcomed and loved by their classmates.

7. Collaborative Communication:

Maintaining open communication between parents, educators, and medical specialists is crucial for safeguarding the student's general well-being and scholastic growth. Regular meetings can assist in discussing difficulties, tracking progress, and making appropriate modifications to the educational plan.

8. Integration of Therapies:

Integrating physical therapy, occupational therapy, and other suitable therapies into the school day can improve the student's physical development and boost their capacity to participate in academic and extracurricular activities.

9. Encouraging Extracurricular Activities:

Encouraging students with progeria to enrol in extracurricular activities can promote social connection, self-confidence, and a sense of belonging. Schools can seek to suit the student's interests and abilities in extracurricular activities, athletics, or creative hobbies.

10. Providing Educational Resources:

Schools should provide teaching tools and materials that adapt to the student's specific requirements and learning styles. Access to audiobooks, extended print materials, or adaptive technologies can facilitate the learning process.

11. Educating Peers:

Educating peers about progeria can increase empathy, minimise misconceptions, and provide a supportive peer environment. Inviting medical professionals or support organisations to speak to the class helps develop understanding and compassion.

12. Home-School Collaboration:

For students with progeria who may encounter frequent medical appointments or hospitalizations, home-school collaboration becomes crucial. Establishing a connection between the student's family and school helps give continuity in learning and promote the student's academic progress despite periods of absence.

13. Self-Advocacy and Empowerment:

Encouraging self-advocacy abilities in students with progeria helps them to articulate their needs, preferences, and concerns effectively. As adolescents mature, greater self-awareness and self-advocacy can help them actively participate in their educational route and foster a feeling of agency.

14. Building Resilience:

Living with progeria takes resilience and adaptability. Schools can play a big part in promoting resilience by fostering a growth attitude, providing coping skills, and recognizing the student's achievements and efforts.

15. Addressing Bullying and Prejudice:

Students with progeria may be susceptible to bullying or prejudice due to their physical appearance and abnormalities. Schools must have clear anti-bullying policies in place and actively address any occurrences of bullying or discrimination to provide a safe and respectful learning environment.

16. Transition Planning:

As students with progeria approach graduation, preparation for post-secondary education or vocational training becomes crucial. Transition planning comprises identifying appropriate opportunities, support services, and accommodations to ensure a smooth transition to adulthood and independence.

17. Peer Support Groups:

Establishing peer support groups can be good for kids with progeria, providing them with the opportunity to connect with others facing similar challenges. Peer support can establish a sense of belonging, lessen feelings of isolation, and increase healthy social interactions.

18. Involvement of Special Education Professionals:

Schools with special education professionals skilled in aiding students with specialised needs can play a significant role in establishing individualised educational plans, giving focused interventions, and promoting positive results for students with progeria.

19. Recognizing and Celebrating Achievements:

Acknowledging the successes and growth of students with progeria, both academically and in other aspects of life, can enhance their self-esteem and motivation. Celebrating their accomplishments creates a pleasant learning experience and encourages their sense of accomplishment.

20. Continued Collaboration with Healthcare Providers:

Regular interaction with healthcare providers is necessary to monitor the student's health, examine any changes in their condition, and alter educational plans as needed. School personnel and medical specialists working together can ensure the student receives thorough care and assistance.

Managing school and education when living with progeria demands a multifaceted strategy that focuses on the student's physical well-being, academic performance, emotional support, and social inclusion.

By offering a collaborative and supportive culture, schools may play a transformational role in the lives of youngsters with progeria, encouraging them to realise their full potential and develop a love of learning that lasts a lifetime.

Through understanding, empathy, and proactive efforts, schools may develop an inclusive and inspiring educational experience for all children, regardless of their specific difficulties and needs.

Chapter 5

<u>NAVIGATING WITH FAMILY</u>

When a family member has progeria, their loved ones play a critical role in delivering support, care, and understanding. Navigating the issues related to progeria takes a cohesive and loving attitude from the entire family. Here are some ways family members can aid when someone in the family has progeria:

1. Educate Themselves About Progeria:
Learning about progeria and understanding its implications is crucial for family members to provide the most possible support. Familiarising yourself with the medical characteristics, symptoms, and probable difficulties of the illness enables family members to be more prepared to

manage the particular requirements of their loved one.

2. Foster an Inclusive and Supportive Environment:

Creating a caring and inclusive home environment is vital for the emotional well-being of the individual with progeria. Family members can offer support, celebrate triumphs, and treat the individual with progeria with the same love and respect as any other family member.

3. Provide Emotional Support:

Living with progeria can be emotionally stressful for the affected individual and their family. Family members can offer emotional support, listen intently, and validate feelings and experiences. Open communication and a non-judgmental attitude can offer a secure space for the individual to share their emotions.

4. Assist with Daily Activities:

Family members can aid with daily chores that may be tougher for the individual with progeria owing to physical limits. Assisting with clothes, grooming, and meal preparation can increase independence while giving practical aid.

5. Facilitate Medical Care and Appointments:

Progeria demands constant medical attention and monitoring. Family members can help arrange medical appointments, manage medications, and contact healthcare providers to ensure the individual's health requirements are addressed.

6. Encourage Independence:

While supplying aid, it's also vital to persuade the individual with progeria to be as autonomous as possible. Encouraging autonomy and offering opportunities for decision-making can promote confidence and self-reliance.

7. Advocate for Inclusivity:

Family members can lobby for inclusivity and understanding within the community, schools, and public places. Raising knowledge about progeria and addressing stereotypes can assist in building a more tolerant environment for their loved ones.

8. Organise Family Activities:

Family activities and outings can bring moments of delight and bonding. Planning activities that are fit for the individual with progeria's physical capabilities guarantees that they may actively participate and feel included.

9. Connect with Support Networks:

Joining support groups or online networks for families affected by progeria can provide crucial resources, knowledge, and a sense of camaraderie with others facing similar problems.

10. Address Sibling Relationships:

Siblings of an individual with progeria may have diverse experiences and sentiments. Family members can foster open communication between siblings, address any concerns they may have, and promote understanding and empathy.

11. Celebrate Achievements:

Acknowledging the accomplishments and milestones of the individual with progeria helps increase their self-esteem and reaffirms their unique talents and abilities.

12. Plan for the Future:

While it can be tough, planning for the future, including end-of-life discussions and preparations, is crucial for the entire family. Having these conversations early on can bring peace of mind and ensure that the individual's desires are respected.

13. Manage Financial and Resource Support:

Progeria might suggest considerable medical expenses, and needing professional treatments and therapies. Family members should work together to study available financial choices, such as health insurance coverage and government aid programs, to ease the financial strain and ensure access to needed medical care.

14. Encourage Social Involvement:

Family members can encourage the individual with progeria to form social connections and friendships. Encouraging involvement in social events, playdates, or support groups can provide crucial social interactions and ease feelings of isolation.

15. Promote Education and Advocacy:

Educating family members about progeria and its repercussions allows them to become champions not only inside the family but also in the wider society. By improving knowledge and addressing misunderstandings, family members can help establish a more inclusive society for individuals with progeria.

16. Engage in Fun and Enriching Activities:

Balancing the trials of life with progeria with intervals of delight and happiness is crucial. Engaging in enjoyable and exciting activities, such as hobbies, arts and crafts, or creative projects, can raise moods and produce lovely family memories.

17. Foster Resilience and Positive Mindset:

Cultivating a resilient and optimistic outlook as a family helps assist in managing the ups and downs of living with progeria. Emphasising strengths, praising accomplishments, and focusing on opportunities rather than limits can boost the family's overall well-being.

18. Support Sibling Bonds:

Nurturing sibling relationships is crucial for developing a stable family dynamic. Family members can encourage siblings to talk honestly, express their thoughts, and give opportunities for positive interactions between siblings.

19. Encourage Personal Growth:

Family members can aid the individual with progeria in following personal interests and aspirations. Encouraging academic achievements, creative hobbies, or sporting pursuits can stimulate personal growth and self-discovery.

20. Seek Professional Guidance:

While family members supply crucial support, receiving professional help from therapists, counsellors, or support organisations can offer extra specialised support and coping techniques for the family as a whole.

21. Adapt & Adjust:

Progeria is a progressive condition, and as the individual's needs vary over time, family members may need to alter their approach and care plans accordingly. Flexibility and agility are key to offering the finest service possible.

Family members play a key position in the life of someone with progeria. Their love, support, and understanding can substantially improve the well-being and quality of life of the individual with progeria.

By working together as a united and caring family, they may help their loved one negotiate the challenges of progeria and create a supportive and inclusive setting where the individual may grow and be treasured for who they are.

Chapter 6

<u>NUTRITION AND LIFESTYLE</u>

Nutritional and lifestyle concerns have a key role in promoting the health and well-being of individuals with progeria.

As a rare and progressive genetic illness, progeria necessitates a holistic approach to nutrition and lifestyle to help control symptoms, optimise growth, and increase the overall quality of life. Here are some essential variables to consider:

1. Balanced and Nutrient-Dense Diet: Providing a balanced and nutrient-dense diet is crucial for persons with progeria. A diet rich in fruits, vegetables, whole grains, lean proteins, and healthy fats can supply crucial vitamins, minerals, and antioxidants that support overall health and growth.

2. Adequate Caloric Intake:

Due to the risk of development failure and decreased muscle mass, it's vital to ensure that persons with progeria acquire enough caloric intake to satisfy their energy needs. This may involve offering smaller, more frequent meals to accommodate diminished appetite or energy consumption.

3. Hydration:

Staying well-hydrated is crucial for persons with progeria, especially if they face difficulty swallowing or absorbing adequate fluids. Encourage frequent water intake and consider offering fluids in easy-to-use containers to facilitate consumption.

4. Supplements:

Depending on the individual's specific nutritional needs, healthcare experts may offer certain supplements, such as calcium and vitamin D for bone health or omega-3 fatty acids for cardiovascular support.

Supplements should be employed on the counsel of healthcare specialists.

5. Caloric Densification:

For patients with progeria who struggle to maintain weight or have trouble eating substantial quantities, caloric densification can be helpful. This comprises blending high-calorie items into meals, such as adding healthy fats (e.g., avocado, nuts) to smoothies or utilising nutrient-rich oils in cooking.

6. Avoiding Processed and Sugary Foods:

Minimising the consumption of processed and sugary meals is crucial for boosting general health and decreasing potential difficulties related to progeria, such as cardiovascular diseases and obesity.

7. Physical Activity and Exercise:

While progeria may limit physical abilities, engaging in correct physical activities and workouts can assist in maintaining muscle strength, flexibility, and overall well-being. Low-impact workouts like stretching, mild yoga, and water aerobics can be good options.

8. Rest and Sleep:

Adequate rest and quality sleep are required for patients with progeria to promote their growth and general health. Creating a tranquil nightly routine and providing a comfortable sleep environment can foster higher sleep quality.

9. Social and Emotional Support:

Providing a caring and nurturing environment can favourably boost emotional well-being. Encourage social interactions, family bonding, and open communication to handle any emotional challenges the individual may have.

10. Reducing Stress:

Managing stress is crucial for patients with progeria, as stress can damage the immune system and overall health. Encouraging relaxation techniques, such as deep breathing exercises or mindfulness practices, can help reduce stress levels.

11. Medical Management:

Regular medical check-ups and vigilant monitoring of health markers are crucial in managing progeria. Collaboration with healthcare professionals, notably dietitians, and specialists, is crucial to personalise interventions to the individual's unique needs.

12. Environmental Considerations:

Ensuring a secure and accessible environment that supports mobility and minimises possible threats is crucial for persons with progeria. Adapting the living place to fit physical limits can increase their freedom and safety.

13. Regular Monitoring of Cardiovascular Health:

Progeria is related to an increased risk of cardiovascular issues, including atherosclerosis. Regular monitoring of blood pressure, cholesterol levels, and heart function is crucial to recognize and address any cardiovascular issues early.

14. Skin Care:

Individuals with progeria may have sensitive skin that is vulnerable to dryness and irritation. Maintaining regular skin care, especially with soft and moisturising solutions, will help avoid skin problems and pain.

15. Dental Care:

Dental health is crucial for general well-being. Regular dental check-ups and basic oral hygiene practices are crucial to avoid dental problems and enhance oral health.

16. Eye Health:

Regular eye examinations are crucial to check for any visual abnormalities or eye-related illnesses that may emerge as a result of progeria.

17. Mental and Emotional Support:

Living with a rare and challenging condition like progeria can be emotionally taxing. Providing mental and emotional support to individuals with progeria and their families is crucial. This may involve counselling, therapy, or participation in support groups to address emotional challenges and encourage coping methods.

18. Family-Centred Care:

Emphasising family-centred care is critical for serving the needs of individuals with progeria comprehensively. Involving family members in the care plan and decision-making process fosters a collaborative approach and ensures that all aspects of the individual's well-being are considered.

19. Safety Precautions:

Taking basic safety precautions is vital to prevent accidents and injuries. Ensuring a safe home environment and offering assistive technologies as needed will help reduce the likelihood of accidents.

20. Collaboration with Support Organisations:

Connecting with support organisations that focus on progeria can provide crucial resources, education, and a sense of community. These groups can offer practical aid, connect families with similar experiences, and keep them updated on the newest research and therapies.

21. Research and Clinical Trials:

Families of persons with progeria may consider participating in research studies or therapeutic trials focused on progeria.

Contributing to medical research can assist in expanding understanding and potential cures for the ailment.

Comprehensive nutritional and lifestyle considerations for people with progeria are crucial for reducing symptoms, preserving optimal health, and increasing overall well-being.

A holistic strategy that incorporates medical management, emotional support, and a safe and caring environment can substantially impact the quality of life for persons living with progeria and their families.

By giving a supportive and inclusive care plan matched to the special needs of each individual, it is possible to improve their quality of life and help them to thrive despite the challenges of progeria.

Chapter 7

<u>CO-OCCURRING CONDITIONS</u>

Progeria is an unusual and complex hereditary disorder that can lead to several difficulties involving multiple systems in the body.

While there is currently no cure for progeria, careful management of its attendant difficulties can assist in improving the individual's quality of life and potentially delay the onset of severe symptoms. Here, we shall study some of the common progeria-related issues and their management:

1. Cardiovascular Complications:

Progeria is intimately related to early ageing of the cardiovascular system, resulting in an increased risk of cardiovascular disorders such as atherosclerosis (narrowing and hardening of the arteries), hypertension (high blood pressure), and heart disease. Management may involve:

- Regular monitoring of blood pressure and cholesterol levels.

- Implementation of a heart-healthy diet, low in saturated fats and abundant in fruits, vegetables, and whole grains.

- Regular physical exercise adapted to the individual's capacities and under medical supervision.

- Medications to treat hypertension or cholesterol levels if necessary.

- Periodic cardiac checkups to assess heart function.

2. Musculoskeletal Complications:

Individuals with progeria may suffer musculoskeletal issues such as joint stiffness, restricted range of motion, and decreased muscle mass. Management may include:

- Physical treatment to develop flexibility, strength, and mobility.

- Assistive equipment includes braces or adaptive tools to support daily activities.

- Encouragement of low-impact workouts to maintain joint health.

- Pain management options, including pharmaceutical and non-pharmacological techniques.

3. Skin Complications:

Progeria can lead to weak and thin skin, making patients susceptible to skin problems like dryness, bruising, and blisters. Management may involve:
Regular use of moisturisers to keep the skin hydrated.

- Protection from excessive sun exposure to avoid skin damage.

- Wound care and early treatment of any injuries.

- Gentle stroking of the skin to limit the chance of bruising or ripping.

4. Respiratory Complications:

Respiratory issues, including respiratory infections and restrictive lung disease, can emerge with progeria. Management may include:

- Regular monitoring of lung function.

- Vaccination against respiratory diseases, as advised by healthcare providers.

- Prompt treatment of respiratory infections to avert complications.

- Encouragement of deep breathing techniques to support lung health.

5. Dental and Oral Complications:

Individuals with progeria may suffer dental issues, such as crowded teeth or delayed tooth eruption. Management may involve:

- Regular dental check-ups and cleanings.

- Orthodontic evaluation and management of dental misalignment.

- Oral hygiene education and actions to prevent dental issues.

6. Growth and Developmental Complications:

Progeria can lead to growth failure and developmental problems. Management may include:

- Monitoring growth metrics periodically.

- Ensuring a balanced and nutrient-dense diet to stimulate growth.

- Providing developmental assistance, including early intervention programs if warranted.

7. Psychological and Emotional Complications:

Living with progeria can present psychological and emotional challenges for affected persons and their families. Management may include:

- Access to mental health support, counselling, or therapy to address emotional well-being.

- Encouragement of open communication within the family and with healthcare practitioners.

- Building a supportive and nurturing atmosphere to enhance emotional resilience.

8. Bone Health Complications:

Individuals with progeria may experience a bone density decrease and an increased risk of fractures. Management may involve:

- Ensuring a suitable amount of calcium and vitamin D through meals and supplements if necessary.

- Encouraging weight-bearing workouts to promote bone health.

- Fall prevention measures to minimise the chance of fractures.

9. Vision and Hearing Complications: Vision and hearing impairments can emerge in some persons with progeria. Management may include:

- Regular eye and hearing checks to detect any changes or problems.

- Providing corrected eyeglasses or hearing aids as needed.

10. Gastrointestinal Complications:

Progeria can damage the gastrointestinal system, leading to issues including constipation or difficulty swallowing. Management may include:

- Adequate hydration and fibre ingestion to assist healthy bowel motions.

- Modification of meal consistency or texture to assist swallowing, as advised by a speech therapist or nutritionist.

11. Endocrine Complications:

Progeria can alter the endocrine system, resulting in hormonal disorders. Management may involve:

- Regular monitoring of hormone levels and proper hormone replacement medication if necessary.

- Consultation with endocrinologists to address any special endocrine-related concerns.

12. Cognitive Complications:

While cognitive deficiencies are rarely a defining characteristic of progeria, some individuals may face moderate cognitive issues. Management may include:

- Providing educational support, including tailored learning plans and accommodations, where appropriate.

- Encouraging cognitive stimulation and engagement in age-appropriate activities to improve cognitive growth.

13. Immunological Complications:

Individuals with progeria may have a weakened immune system, leaving them more susceptible to infections. Management may involve:

- Ensuring compliance with recommended immunizations to guard against infectious illnesses.

- Implementing infection control procedures to limit the danger of exposure to microorganisms.

14. Social Inclusion and Emotional Support:

Addressing the psychological components of progeria is crucial for promoting general well-being. Management may include:

- Encouraging social inclusion and offering opportunities for social contacts and peer support.

- Offering emotional aid to both those with progeria and their families to cope with the hardships of the condition.

15. Pain Management:

Some patients with progeria may suffer pain, either owing to problems or other medical reasons. Management may involve: Identifying and addressing the source of suffering through medical examinations.

Implementing pain management alternatives, which may involve medicines, physical therapy, or relaxation techniques.

16. Preventive Measures:

Proactive measures can play a major role in reducing progeria-related disorders. Family members and healthcare practitioners may consider:

- Promoting a healthy lifestyle that includes a balanced diet, regular exercise, and suitable relaxation.

- Regular health check-ups to watch for potential effects and resolve issues immediately.

- Creating a safe and accessible living environment to decrease the likelihood of accidents or injury.

17. Research and Clinical Trials:

Engaging in research projects or clinical trials concentrating on progeria can contribute to growing information and new therapy options for the condition. Participation in research can aid future generations of individuals with progeria.

18. Family Education and Empowerment:

Providing families with a thorough education about progeria and its accompanying issues encourages them to be active partners in their loved one's treatment. Family members who are well-educated can make informed choices and advocate for their loved one's needs effectively.

19. Palliative Care:

In some instances, patients with progeria may require palliative treatment to control symptoms and improve their quality of life. Palliative care focuses on treating pain and discomfort, fostering emotional well-being, and enhancing the overall quality of life.

20. End-of-Life Care:

In circumstances when progeria substantially diminishes life expectancy, end-of-life care becomes crucial. Providing compassionate and thorough end-of-life care includes addressing medical, emotional, and spiritual needs and preserving the individual's comfort and dignity.

Controlling progeria-related disorders demands a multidisciplinary and personalised strategy that addresses the particular needs of each person.

Collaborating with healthcare providers, getting essential medicines and therapies, and building a supportive family environment are key components in enhancing the well-being and quality of life of individuals with progeria.

With continuing research and an emphasis on holistic treatment, discoveries in managing progeria-related diseases continue to grow, giving hope and improved results for affected individuals and their families.

Chapter 8

<u>MEDICAL TREATMENT OPTIONS</u>

Medical care of progeria seeks to address the multiple symptoms and effects connected with the condition, improve the individual's quality of life, and boost overall well-being.

While there is presently no cure for progeria, a multidisciplinary strategy involving medical specialists, therapists, and supportive care is crucial for providing comprehensive management. Here are some main components of medical care for patients with progeria:

1. Regular Medical Check-ups:
Consistent medical surveillance is necessary to track the evolution of progeria and detect any effects early. Regular check-ups with

paediatricians or professionals experienced with progeria are recommended to monitor growth, development, and overall health.

2. Cardiovascular Management:

As cardiovascular issues are common in progeria, continuous monitoring and care are essential. This may require regular blood pressure checks, lipid profile monitoring, and cardiac exams, including echocardiograms, to examine heart function.

3. Medications:

Medications may be advised to manage certain symptoms or effects connected with progeria. For instance, medications may be used to regulate blood pressure, reduce cholesterol levels, or address bone density issues.

4. Pain Management:

Individuals with progeria may have difficulty owing to musculoskeletal difficulties or other linked illnesses. Pain management methods, including over-the-counter or prescription medicines, physical therapy, and relaxation techniques, could help minimise discomfort.

5. Physical Therapy:

Physical therapy is a crucial component of progeria management. Physical therapists can develop tailored exercise plans to promote mobility, flexibility, and strength. These exercises can help patients with progeria keep independence and reduce the threat of joint contractures.

6. Nutritional Support:

Nutrition plays a crucial role in reducing progeria-related disorders. A well-balanced diet, including proper calories, nutrients, and hydration, is necessary to support growth, bone health, and general well-being.

7. Bone Health:

Promoting bone health is vital in progeria care. Ensuring a suitable intake of calcium and vitamin D, as well as encouraging weight-bearing activities, can assist in maintaining bone density and minimise the chance of fractures.

8. Dental Care:

Regular dental check-ups and dental treatment are crucial for keeping oral health and treating any dental issues that may occur in individuals with progeria.

9. Immunizations:

Vaccinations are important for patients with progeria to safeguard against preventable infectious infections. Following advised vaccine schedules helps boost their immune system.

10. Respiratory Support:

Individuals with progeria may require respiratory support if they develop restrictive lung disease or respiratory difficulties. This may need employing support devices or respiratory therapy.

11. Genetic Counselling:

Genetic counselling is crucial for families affected by progeria. Genetic counsellors can provide information about the illness, its inheritance pattern, and family planning alternatives.

12. Palliative Care and Supportive Measures:

Palliative care focuses on reducing symptoms and delivering comfort and support for patients with progeria. It treats pain, emotional well-being, and overall quality of life.

13. Mental and Emotional Support:

Emotional well-being is vital for individuals with progeria and their families. Access to mental health care, counselling, or therapy can be effective in resolving emotional challenges and cultivating coping mechanisms.

14. Surgical Interventions:

In rare cases, surgical therapies may be needed to address specific concerns connected to progeria. For instance, orthopaedic operations may be performed to repair joint abnormalities or reduce discomfort caused by skeletal defects. Surgical procedures can also address cardiovascular diseases, such as repairing heart valve abnormalities.

15. Supportive Devices and Adaptive Equipment:

Depending on the individual's needs, the use of supportive devices and adaptive equipment can facilitate everyday living and movement. These may include braces, walkers, adapted seats, or assistance devices geared to aid in various activities.

16. Communication Strategies:

Individuals with progeria may face communication challenges, especially if they exhibit speech or hearing impairments. Implementing different communication methods, such as sign language or assistive communication equipment, can increase effective communication and expression.

17. Clinical Trials and Experimental Therapies:

In recent years, clinical research and experimental drugs have appeared to evaluate potential therapies for progeria. Participation in these studies helps patients with progeria and their families to contribute to medical research and maybe acquire breakthrough therapies.

18. Education and Advocacy:

Education regarding progeria, both within the medical community and the public, is crucial to promote awareness, improve early detection, and enhance care for affected patients. Advocacy efforts can lead to increased funding for research, better access to resources, and improved care options.

19. Multidisciplinary Care Team:

Providing comprehensive medical management for progeria requires a coordinated strategy with a multidisciplinary care team. This team may comprise paediatricians, geneticists, cardiologists, endocrinologists, physical therapists, occupational therapists, nutritionists, and mental health specialists.

20. Clinical Care Guidelines:

The Progeria Research Foundation (PRF) and other organisations have published clinical care recommendations to assist healthcare practitioners in managing individuals with progeria effectively. These guidelines offer evidence-based advice for numerous aspects of progeria care.

21. Proactive Monitoring and Research:

Progeria is a complex ailment, and continuous study is required to further understand the disease's processes and potential remedies. Continual monitoring of advancements in progeria research can impact medical care and enhance the outlook for affected individuals.

22. Family Support Groups:

Joining support groups specifically designed for relatives of individuals with progeria can be beneficial. These organisations create a sense of community, a platform for exchanging experiences, and chances for emotional support and resource sharing.

23. Personalised Care Plans:

Recognizing that progeria can show differently in each individual, tailored treatment regimens are essential to suit distinct requirements and challenges. Care plans should be frequently assessed and updated as necessary to match changes in the individual's condition.

In conclusion, the medical management of progeria comprises a comprehensive and interdisciplinary approach, addressing multiple problems and supporting the general well-being of affected patients.

Proactive monitoring, therapeutic interventions, and a supportive care team can drastically enhance the quality of life for individuals with progeria and empower them to thrive despite the barriers offered by the condition.

Collaborative efforts among healthcare professionals, persons with progeria, and their families, coupled with ongoing research and activism, play a critical role in expanding knowledge and care for those touched by progeria.